# THE ULTIMATE GUIDE TO CHARCOAL TEETH WHITENING:
## HOW TO TAKE YOUR SMILE TO THE NEXT LEVEL-THE NATURAL WAY!



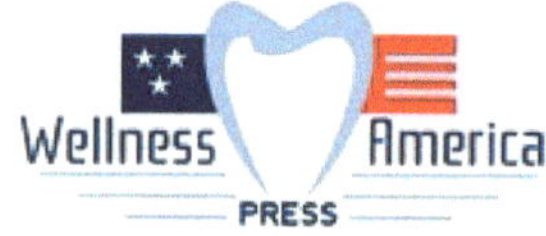


## Disclaimer

This publication is designed to provide accurate and authoritative information r garding the subject matter covered. The author does not accept liability for incident or consequential damages resulting from the use of the information in this book. Th book is designed to assist with exploring various options for improving your smi with cosmetic and general dentistry. It does not make decisions for the individual b provides a range of options to be considered. No responsibility is accepted for ar liability resulting from the actions of any parties involved.

# Table of Contents

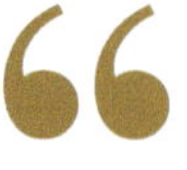

# What People Are Saying About Dr. Catrise Austin & Her Smile Transforming Treatments

"Thank you for aiding in my smile. I love and appreciate your work and dedication!"

**- PAULA ABDUL**
*American Idol host and Grammy-award winning singer*

"Working with Dr. Austin has been the best experience I have had with any dentist ever. Her work is beautiful! Since working with Dr. Austin, I have gotten constant compliments about my teeth. I feel confident and enthused to smile. She's the freshest!"

**- COMMON**
*Grammy Award Winning Rapper and Actor*

"Dr. Austin is a passionate voice for consumers. She understands the whole person she works with – both the visual benefits of cosmetic dentistry and the improved self-esteem it can provide."

**- MICHELE KLINGENSMITH**
*Aquafresh Senior Brand Manager, GlaxoSmith Kline Consumer Healthcare*

"Want to know what it takes to get your smile ready for the red carpet? Dr. Austin! She is a rare talent in her field; her dental expertise is matched by her compassionate understanding of her clients' personal and professional needs, especially anyone in the television, film, music or fashion industries where having a beautiful smile gives you a competitive edge."

**- JACQUELINE J. GONZALEZ**
*Executive Director, National Academy of Television Arts and Sciences, New York*

"Well I'm not a celebrity and Dr. Catrise Austin was my choice. The way I stumbled across her practice was definitely something that was destined because I needed a health professional with compassion for their patients because without them who would the health professional be. It's not all about being of a certain social status it's about hardworking people like me that put their trust and hard earned money into their health. Thank you."

**- ANONYMOUS**

## INTRODUCTION

# Can Activated Charcoal Really Whiten Teeth?

The idea of whitening teeth with charcoal can seem counter-intuitive at first. Charcoal is dark in color and when you begin brushing your teeth with activated charcoal your teeth and gums turn black.

In fact, when you use activated charcoal for the first time your teeth and gums can become so black that your mouth may look a little scary or creepy to you ... and you may naturally begin to wonder if you have made a terrible mistake.

After all, drop charcoal on a tile floor and it will permanently stain the grout. So shouldn't activated charcoal also stain your teeth – making them darker instead of lighter?

Fortunately, the answer to that question is "no" and we'll go into greater detail as to exactly why that is later in this book.

For now, just know that activated charcoal is a powerful purifying agent that absorbs impurities - like stains on your teeth that are caused by coffee, soda, wine, cigarettes and other things.

It really can make your teeth whiter and brighter and it does it without using any harsh chemicals like some man-made teeth whiteners use. Activated charcoal is completely natural. In fact, it is often used by hospitals to treat poisoning victims because it quickly binds to toxins and then removes them from the body.

Using activated charcoal to whiten teeth can be a great way to avoid th
expense (and possible discomfort) associated with other teeth whitenir
methods.

In this book, we are going to take a closer look at using activated charco
to whiten teeth. We are going to explain how the process works and wha
results you can expect.

We are also going to:

- Answer frequently asked questions so that you can better dete
  mine if using activated charcoal is right for you
- Look at how to select the right activated charcoal powder, incluc
  ing what ingredients to look for
- Explain the benefits of using activated charcoal
- Reveal how to keep your teeth white after using activated charcoa
- And much more

So let's get started.

# CHAPTER 1

# What Causes Teeth to Stain?

To begin our journey on the road to a brighter smile, it's important for you to first understand the causes of teeth discoloration.

WHAT CAUSES TEETH TO STAIN?

Stained teeth aren't something to be ashamed of; it happens to the best of us. You see, most of us start out with sparkling white teeth. But over time the color of our teeth may discolor for a variety of reasons. There are natural and environmental reasons why teeth stain; then there are reasons related to different food and beverages.  Let's review some of these causes.

The Most Common Causes of Teeth Stains

## Cause #1: Age

Just as our hair changes to grey as we get older as an indication of age, the same thing happens with teeth. As you age, the outer layer or your teeth slowly wears away and your teeth appear more yellow.  In addition, what you eat, combined with your age, can cause even additional discolorations of the teeth.  For instance, if you drink coffee daily and smoke for fifty years know that your teeth will be far more yellow or brown than someone of the same age who refrains from smoking or consuming coffee.

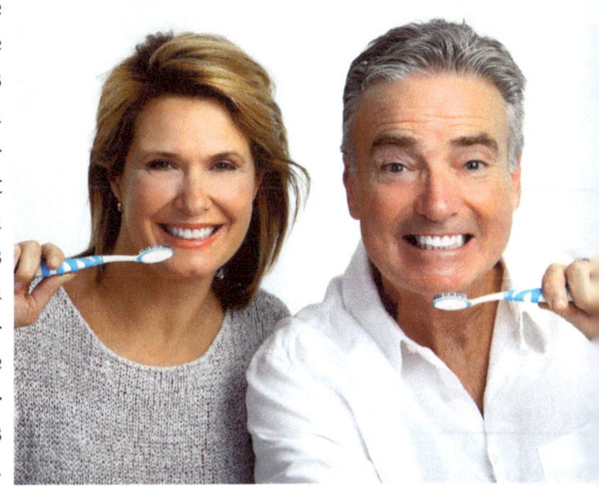

The good news is, no matter what age you are, you can easily improving t[...] color of your smile. Sure, teenagers and those in their twenties will have [...] easier time whitening their teeth, but an older person can make a drama[...] impact with a series of whitening efforts. Plus, a whiter and more confide[...] smile can make you appear younger!

## Cause #2: The Color You're Born With

Did you know the color of teeth you're born with might impact how yo[...] teeth appear throughout your life? It's true! Since birth, we're all equipp[...] with an inborn tooth color that ranges from white, to yellow, to y[...] low-brown, to brown-grey. This color can intensify with time. Teeth th[...] have white and yellow tones respond best to teeth whitening treatmen[...] Brown-grey shades aren't as easy to whiten as the yellow-brown shades. [...] teeth whitening is not 100% effective for eliminating your discolored teet[...] additional dental procedures like porcelain veneers may be needed.

## Cause #3: Eating habits

Eating and drinking highly-pigmented foods is one of the common wa[...] that teeth get discolored over time. Red wine, coffee, tea, dark colas, da[...] berries, and other deeply-colored beverages and foods cause considerab[...] staining over the years. The general rule of thumb that I share with [...] patients in New York is:

> **"** *If what you eat or drink will stain a white T-Shirt,*
> *it will stain your teeth!*

I know that health gurus recommend drinking a glass of red wine for hea[...] health, and eating superfoods like blueberries offer huge health benefi[...] The big tradeoff over time may be a change in the appearance of your teet[...] But don't worry, you'll later learn tips on how to keep your teeth white [...] matter what you eat!

## Cause #4: Tobacco Use

Hey if you are a smoker, I'm not here to preach to you. You already kno[...] about the overall health implications of smoking and (Yes!) you shou[...] really consider quitting to live longer. But as your expert dentist, I ha[...] to talk about how smoking affects your mouth and the color of your teet[...]

The nicotine and tar in tobacco products like cigarettes, pipes, and cigars can do a number on your teeth! From my years of observing smoker's stains in my office, these stains not only accumulate quickly if you use tobacco frequently, the stains are usually pretty severe and challenging to remove.

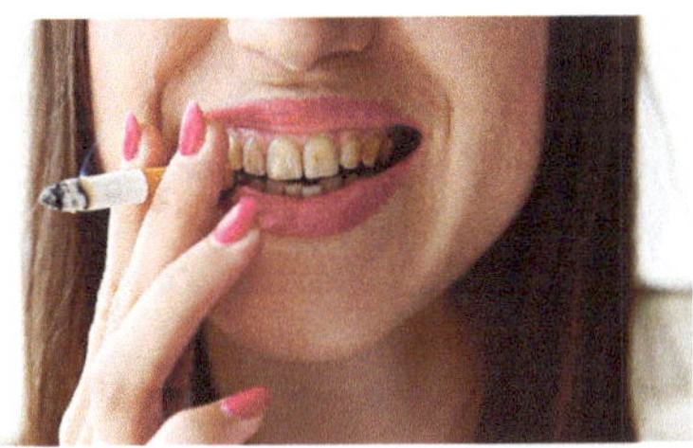

## Cause #5: Medication

Many times stained teeth are the result of the use of prescribed medications. Tetracycline and doxycycline are two antibiotics commonly known to discolor teeth, especially when they are given to children before the age of 8 (when the permanent teeth are still developing). Certain mouth rinses containing chlorhexidine and other chloride rinses that your dentist may prescribe to fight gum disease will also stain teeth. Ask your dentist to explain the risks vs. benefits when prescribing these rinses. These particular stains usually stain the teeth distinctively a brown or grey color with dark lines/striations in the teeth. If your teeth are discolored as a result of using one of these medications

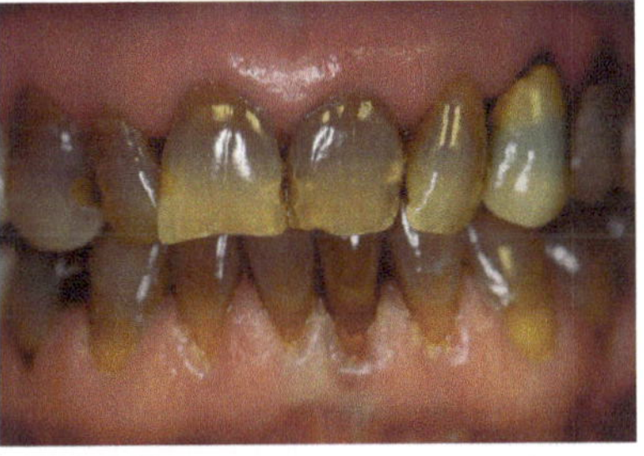

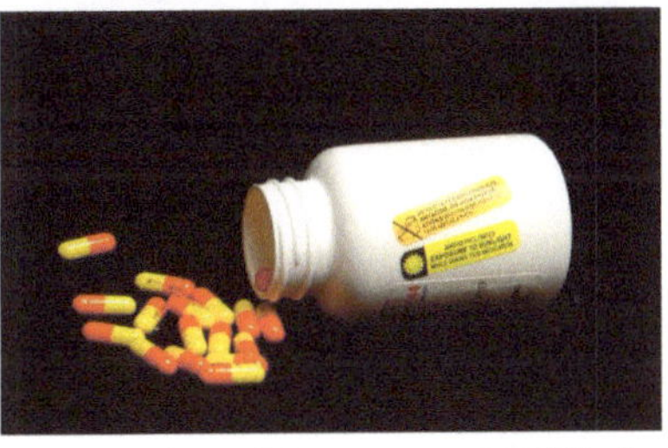

currently or in the past, the good news is your dental insurance MAY help you pay for your whitening treatment!

## Cause #6: Enamel Erosion and Cracking

You should also know that consuming acidic foods and drinks can promote staining of the teeth. The acidity of coffee, wine, lemons, oranges (to name a few) will contribute to enamel erosion. When enamel erodes, pigmented molecules called chromogens are able to latch on to the tooth's enamel easier, thus leading to tooth staining.

Micro-cracking is what happens when you grind or clinch your teeth. This activity, usually brought on by stress, will cause your teeth to pick up stain.

In addition, bad habits like ice chewing, pen or chewing, and using your teeth to open bottles can cause micro-cracks that can pick up stains.

## Tooth Discoloration: The Two Types of Tooth Stains

There are two categories of teeth staining: extrinsic staining and intrinsic staining.

**Extrinsic stains** appear only on the outer enamel surface of the teeth as a result of exposure to dark colored beverages, foods, and tobacco. Superficial extrinsic stains are minor and can be removed pretty easy at home with activated charcoal or other professional dental treatments. It's important to understand that persistent extrinsic stains can penetrate into the layer below the enamel and become ingrained if they are not dealt with early. The key is to remove extrinsic stains as soon as they become visible.

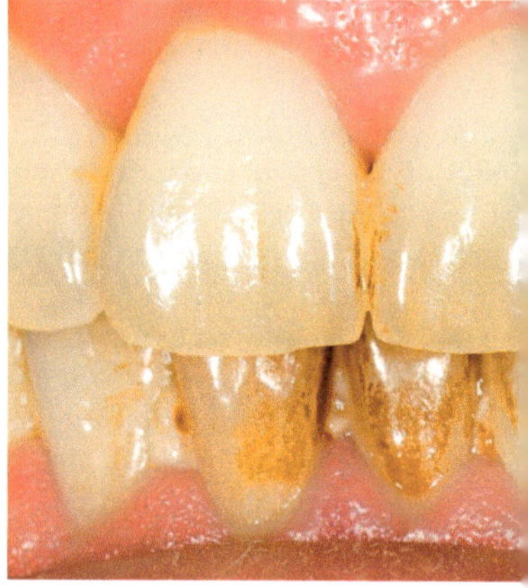

*Extrinsic stain*

**Intrinsic stains** are deeper stains that form below the enamel layer of teeth. These stains result from trauma, aging, excessive exposure to fluoride or tetracycline during tooth formation. It is a myth that intrinsic stains are too resistant to be corrected by bleaching. However, depending on the color and severity, some deep-set intrinsic stains can be removed with supervised take-home teeth whitening products or in office professional whitening. If teeth whitening does not successfully remove your intrinsic stains, your dentist may suggest upgrading to alternate treatments like porcelain veneers or porcelain crowns to permanently mask the discoloration.

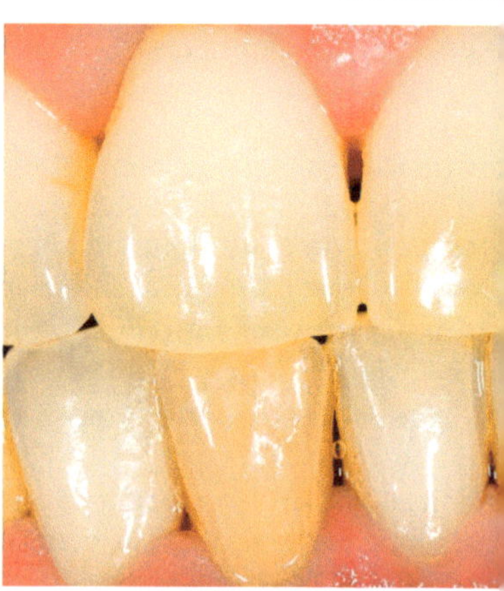

*Intrinsic stain*

# CHAPTER 2

# Whitening Teeth With Activated Charcoal

If you are on social media (and who isn't these days) then you probably have seen a video of someone whitening their teeth with activated charcoal or, at least, read a message about this method and its results.

Mainstream media has also been covering the trend – publications including Men's Health, Shape Magazine, Paper Magazine, the Business Insider, The Fresno Bee, the Mercury News and many more have all had articles about whitening teeth with activated charcoal.

Many celebrities – including Ferne McCann, Marnie Simpson, Vicky Pattison, Pete Wicks, Nicole Scherzinger and Drake – credit activated charcoal for giving them their pearly whites.

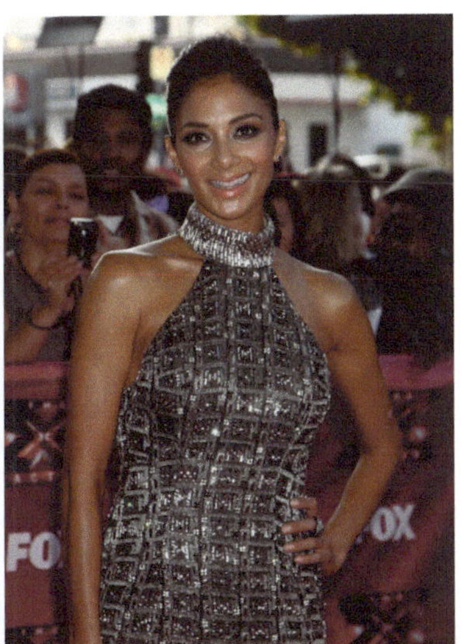

Scherzinger, of The Pussycat Dolls fame, told the Daily Mail:

> *I'd much rather brush my teeth with coal, which I've done. That's even better. Makes your teeth whiter.*

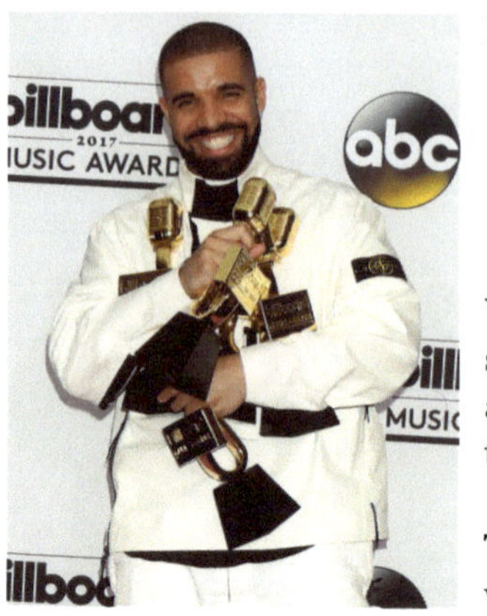

Drake told Paper Magazine:

> I brush with activated charcoal before any club night where I will see baddies know dattttttttt.

Whitening teeth with activated charcoal soaring in popularity and many people toda are wondering if you really can whiten you teeth this way.

The short answer is "yes you can." Here what you need to know:

## What exactly is activated charcoal?

While it's not the charcoal that you fire up your grill with, it is very close to that substance.

Activated charcoal is created by using a gas to heat up charcoal. This process creates large pours in the mineral which are then capable of trapping chemicals. This is why activated charcoal is so absorbent and can be used by hospitals to treat food poisoning and other types of poisoning incidents.

The activated charcoal binds to the toxins and then since the body does not absorb charcoal, the toxins are passed safely out of the body.

Activated charcoal is also used to treat intestinal gas and cholestasis during pregnancy. It can also be used to lower cholesterol.

When used to whiten teeth, the charcoal binds to toxins in the mouth and removes them – this includes stains on the teeth as well as bacteria that can cause cavities and gum disease.

That's right, activated charcoal is actually good for the mouth!

Let's take a closer look at how it works:

The activated charcoal's pores, which we discussed previously, bind with surface stains, food particles and plaque on the teeth and remove them as you rinse the charcoal out of your mouth.

The result is whiter, brighter teeth. However, please keep in mind that the degree of whiteness and brightness achieved will vary by person. Activated charcoal also may not change the color of teeth that are deeply stained or naturally yellowing. As we said previously it is more of a treatment for extrinsic stains instead of intrinsic stains.

So let me say that again: Activated charcoal is more for the removal of surface stains – a job which it is excellent at.

Is activated charcoal safe?

Yes, food-grade, activated charcoal is safe to ingest but there are a few things to keep in mind.

>    **1.** Ingesting too much charcoal can cause constipation and block mineral absorption. It can also cause dehydration. Simply brushing with activated charcoal and spitting it out should not cause any health problems.
>
>    **2.** You should brush gently with activated charcoal, the abrasiveness of the mineral can damage teeth if it is vigorously scrubbed against them.

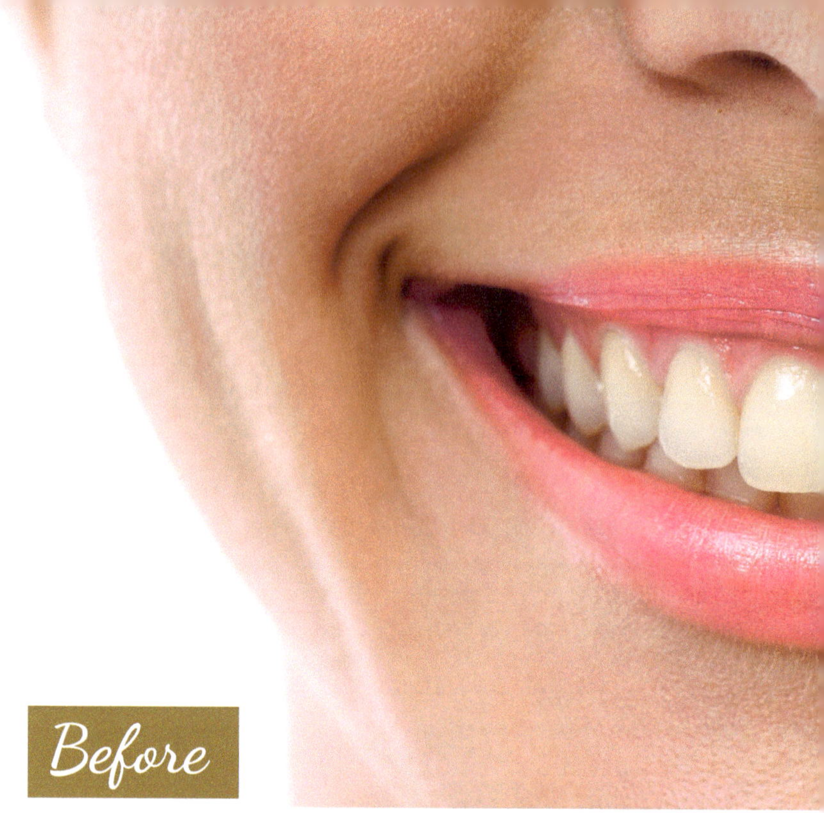

14

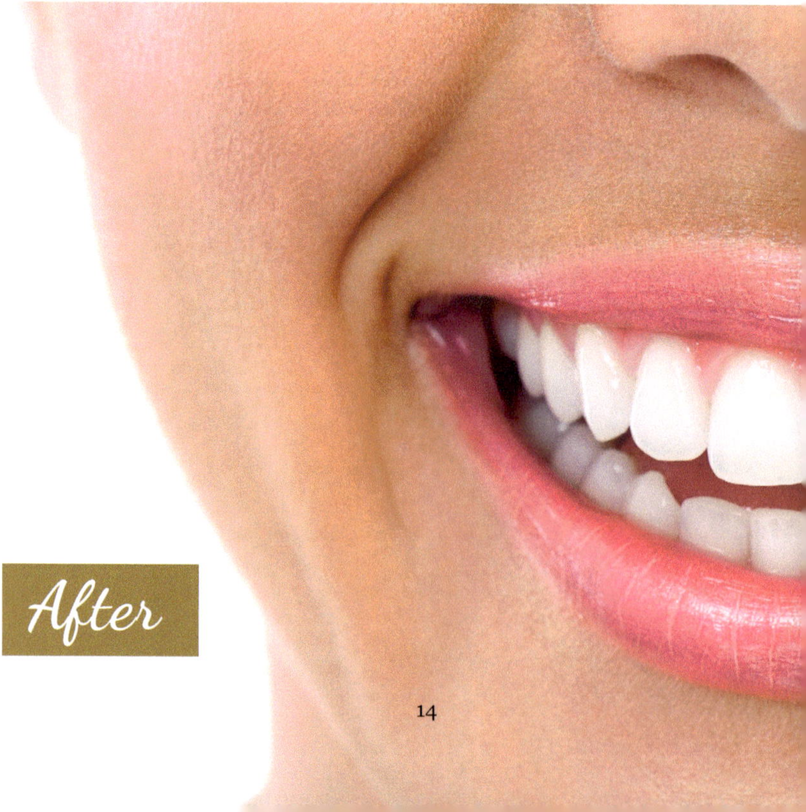

CHAPTER 3

# How to Use Activated Charcoal to Whiten Your Teeth

Activated charcoal makes whitening teeth as easy as 1, 2, 3.

**1.** Simply wet a toothbrush and dip it into the activated charcoal powder.

**2.** Next brush your teeth like normal for 1 to 2 minutes.

**3.** Rinse thoroughly. The nonabrasive formula binds to stains on teeth and gently removes them - making your teeth whiter and brighter over time.

Most who use this method of teeth whitening are surprised the first time they try it because when all the black in their mouth washes away their teeth immediately feel extremely clean and smooth.

After just a few uses, many begin to notice their teeth getting whiter – but again results vary by individual.

A few things to remember:

- Activated charcoal can be extremely messy as it is a fine powder that is easy to spill. As a result, when opening the lid on your activated charcoal bottle go slowly and be extremely careful.
- You should also use a small amount of powder on your tooth brush - with activated charcoal a little definitely goes a long way.

- Activated charcoal stains! So you may want to use a separa[te] toothbrush for it.
- Don't get freaked out when your mouth and teeth look black! Th[is] is natural and will rinse away when you are finished brushin[g]. Then your teeth will feel much smoother and cleaner.

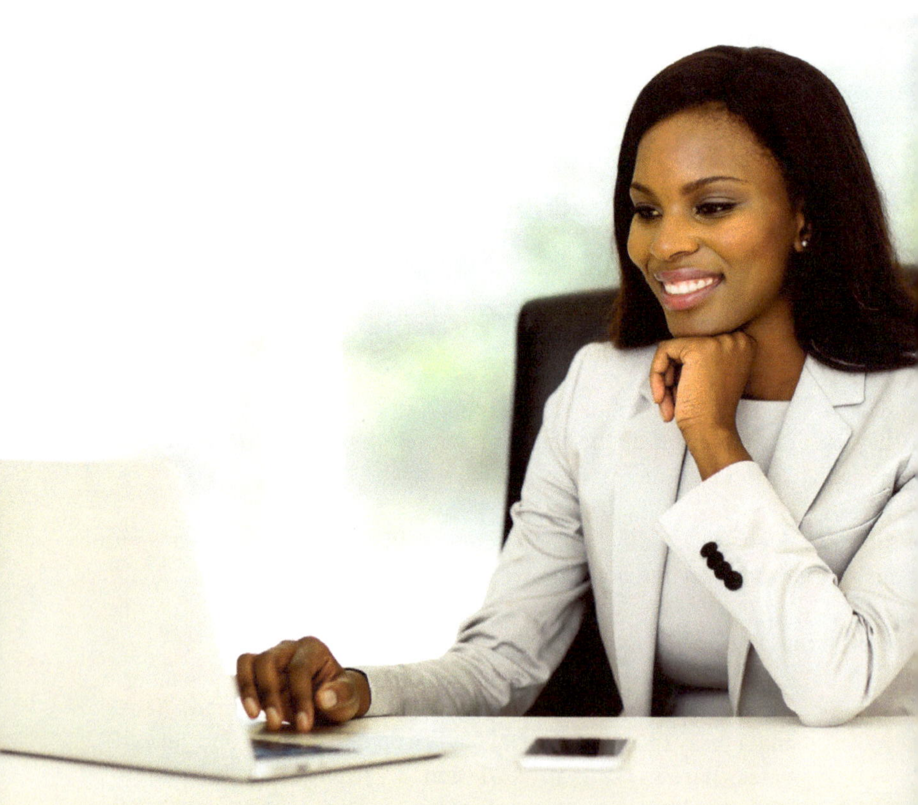

# CHAPTER 4

# How to Select an Activated Charcoal Teeth Whitening Powder

As is the case with any type of supplement there are activated charcoal teeth whitening powders that are better than others.

In this chapter we are going to tell you what to look for when selecting an activated charcoal powder.

What to look for:

> **1.** Look for a product that is made from organic coconut sources instead of hardwood or, even worse, a petroleum base. For example, do not use leftover charcoal from a barbecue grill or charcoal from a bag of charcoal briquettes to try to whiten your teeth. Also do not use charcoal pencils or other types of charcoal. Charcoal from organic coconut is the best and safest choice.

> **2.** Look for a product that contains other natural teeth whitening substances, like Organic Orange Seed Oil and Sodium Bicarbonate, which are both effective teeth whiteners. These substances in the right proportions will combine with the activated charcoal to enable you to take your smile to a whole new level!

> **3.** Look for a product that contains mint. Charcoal is generally odorless and tasteless but an activated charcoal teeth whitener with mint will have a pleasant flavor, no bad after-taste and can also freshen and improve your breath.

**4.** Look for a product that is made in the USA and by a comp
ny you can trust. Unfortunately, many companies today are ju
out to make money and cut corners to improve their profits. As
result their products may contain inferior ingredients or be man
factured poorly. Look for a product that contains only the highe
quality natural ingredients and that is manufactured in a state-o
the art facility.

We recommend:

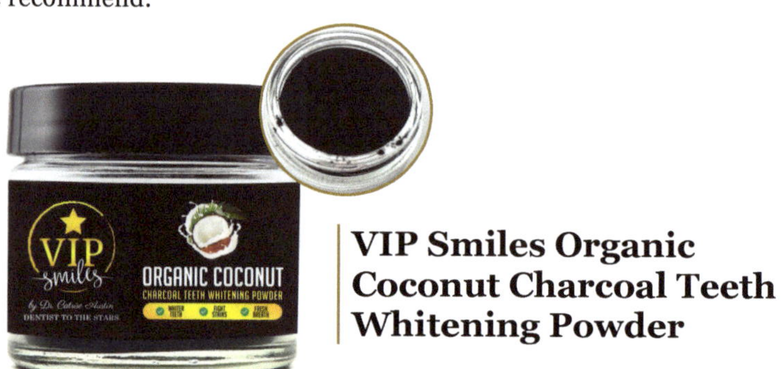


## VIP Smiles Organic Coconut Charcoal Teeth Whitening Powder

This powder is 2 FL OZ Food Grade Activated Charcoal which brighte
teeth, is easy on the gums, is mint flavored and has no bad after-taste.

# CHAPTER 5

# What Are the Benefits of Using Activated Charcoal as a Teeth Whitener?

- You'll avoid harsh whitening products that can irritate your gums and make your teeth sensitive

- Activated charcoal naturally whitens teeth - removing stains caused by coffee, soda, wine, cigarettes and more

- Activated charcoal made from organic coconut sources is food grade and can be ingested. You can use it daily to clean teeth ... or periodically to remove stains

- Activated charcoal powder is also affordable. You can get it at a fraction of the cost of many professional teeth whitening options

- Activated charcoal doesn't just remove stains. It also targets plaque helping to prevent periodontal disease ... and bad breath! Get a product with mint for better taste and even fresher breath

- Activated charcoal is easy to use. Simply wet a toothbrush and dip it into the powder. Then brush your teeth like normal for 1 to 2 minutes before rinsing thoroughly. The nonabrasive formula binds to stains on teeth and gently removes them - making your teeth whiter and brighter over time.

- Some activated charcoal formulas have added whitening power. These formulas contain natural ingredients like Organic Orange Seed Oil and Sodium Bicarbonate, which are also effective teeth whiteners. These substances combine with the activated charcoal to enable you to take your smile to a whole new level!

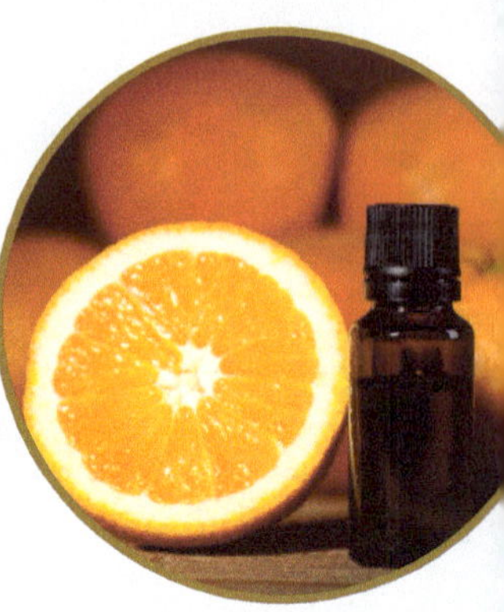

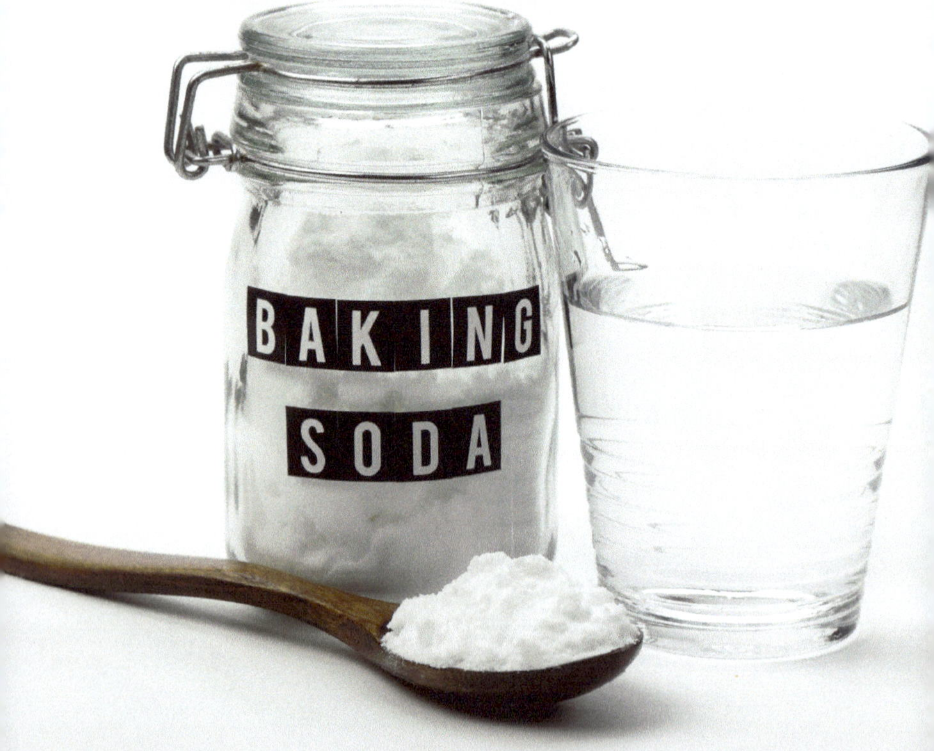

# CHAPTER 6

# Frequently Asked Questions

In this chapter we have compiled and answered some of the most frequently asked questions about using activated charcoal to whiten teeth.

**Do charcoal teeth whitening products stain crowns or porcelain veneers?**
No. The great news is that porcelain crowns and porcelain veneers simply do not stain or change colors no matter what it comes in contact with, including charcoal teeth whitening products. Once you select the color of your dental work, it will remain the same color until it has to be replaced.

**Do charcoal teeth whitening products remove calcium from the teeth?**
Charcoal teeth whitening powder does not decalcify the teeth. It simply absorbs impurities.

**Is charcoal too abrasive for teeth?**
The truth of the matter is that that because this a new dental trend, there hasn't been enough studies done to confirm how abrasive charcoal on teeth. The key however is to choose the best grade of fine charcoal powder to brush with. The finer charcoal powders are usually more expensive, but will be safer.

**What type of teeth stains does the charcoal work on?**
Charcoal teeth whitening powders will only work on surface stains, stains that bind to the outer enamel layer of the teeth. Examples of surface stains include: coffee, tea, and smoker's stains, those from drinks

like coffee and tea. The absorbent properties of the charcoal just pull tl
stains from the surface of the teeth. Don't expect charcoal teeth white
ing powders to work on teeth that naturally have a deep yellow, grey,
brown tone; or teeth that have been discolored from antibiotics or oth
internal problems. For these types of discolorations, you'll need to bi
a professional strength teeth whitening product with a teeth whitenii
agent like hydrogen peroxide or try a 1 hour in-office Teeth Whitenii
session with a dental professional. If your teeth do not respond well
teeth whitening, then the next step is to consider getting porcelain v
neers to totally mask those resistant discolorations.

**What is the difference between products that remove surfa
stains and hydrogen peroxide containing products that whi
en the teeth?**

Not all teeth whiteners are created equal. Surface stains live on the ou
er enamel layer of the teeth and can generally be removed with tootl
paste or surface whitening treatments like the charcoal teeth whitenii
powder. Deeper stains that are below the enamel surface usually requi
a stronger, professional strength teeth whitening agent like hydroge
peroxide. I recommend doing a tooth color analysis with a tooth coli
shade guide at home or with your dentist so that you can gauge whe
your teeth are on the color spectrum and which teeth whitening produ
would be best to brighten your smile.

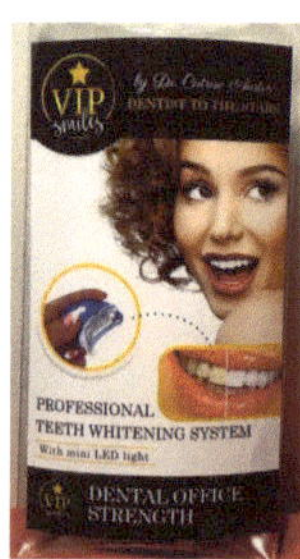
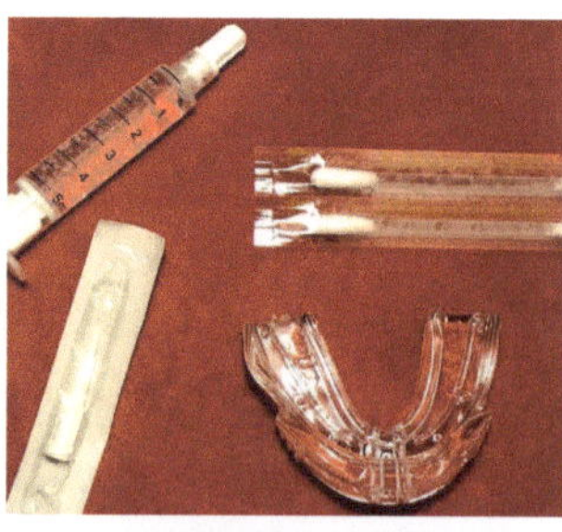

*VIP Smiles
Professional Take home
teeth whitening kit*

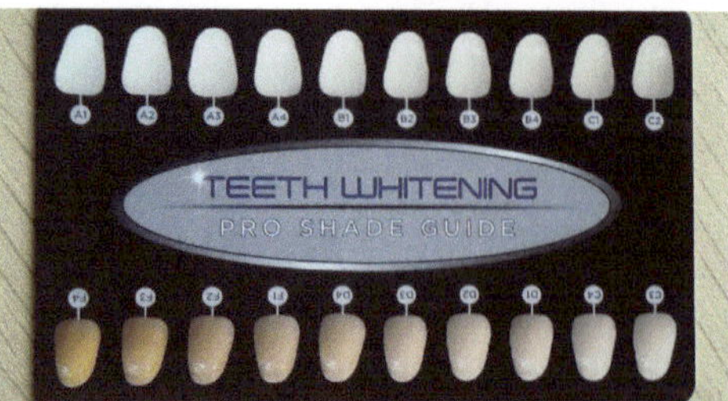

*VIP Smiles
Teeth Whitening
Shade Guide*

**How does activated charcoal teeth whitening work?**
The secret is that activated charcoal is highly absorbent. In fact, activated charcoal is so absorbent that hospitals keep it on hand as a "go to" treatment for poisoning cases because it safely remove toxins from the body. Well the same concept works for whitening the teeth. It pulls bacteria, toxins and stains making the teeth whiter as a result.

**What type of toothpaste should I use while using the charcoal teeth whitening product?**
You can continue to use your toothpaste brand of choice. I recommend using fluoride toothpastes to help fight cavities, but if you prefer keeping it natural feel free to use the natural brand that makes you happy. Although charcoal will detoxify your mouth, I wouldn't recommend using charcoal as a complete substitute for toothpaste.

**Is charcoal teeth whitening safe?**
As far as safety goes, the activated charcoal powder is safe to use in your mouth and ingest. It's even sold in health food stores in a tablet form. As with using baking soda, you have to be mindful that it is abrasive and if not used with the proper toothbrush or with the proper brushing technique it could potentially harm the enamel of the teeth.

**What type of toothbrush should I use with the activated charcoal?**
You can use a soft bristled toothbrush with charcoal infused toothbrush bristles along with your toothpaste of choice.

**Is activated charcoal teeth whitening powder gluten free?**
Yes, not only is it gluten free, it's also kosher, and contains no GMO.

**Is it difficult to get all the charcoal out of your mouth?**
Yes, it can be. We recommend rinsing thoroughly and then brushing your teeth again with a regular toothpaste to get rid of all the charcoal. You may also want to floss.

**Should I brush my teeth before using activated charcoal?**
You can but you certainly don't have to. Remember, activated charcoal

binds with toxins, bacteria and plaque in your mouth and removes
– leaving your teeth to feel even cleaner and smoother. So why not l
the full cleaning power of the activated charcoal work by not brushir
beforehand?

**Does activated charcoal strengthen your teeth?**
It doesn't necessarily make your teeth stronger per se but it does he
make them healthier, which in turn could help them grow stronger. A
tivated charcoal removes plaque and bacteria that can cause gingivitis.

**Is it better to get a formula with just activated charcoal or wit
other natural ingredients?**
We recommend a formula that contains activated charcoal and a fe
natural ingredients like Organic Orange Seed Oil and Sodium Bicarbo
ate for added whitening power. You never know which substance is g
ing to work best for you and by having a few of the best in one produ
you will increase your chances of getting the whitening results you war

**How do you use activated charcoal?**
We recommend wetting a toothbrush and dipping it into activated cha
coal powder. Then brush your teeth like normal for 1 to 2 minutes befo
rinsing thoroughly.

**How soon will I notice results?**
Results vary by individual but many report brighter teeth that fe
smoother and cleaner after the first use. If you don't notice results in
mediately, keep using the product and we are confident you will begin
notice results soon.

**Is it safe to use activated charcoal with crowns? Could th
grains get under the crown?**
It is safe to use with crowns. A properly glued crown won't allow ar
grains to get underneath it.

**Is the activated charcoal gritty?**
It can feel a little gritty in your mouth but it is not generally "overly gri
ty." Do not vigorously scrub your teeth with the activated charcoal

avoid being abrasive to your teeth. Instead brush normally or even gently.

**If I stop using the charcoal powder will my teeth go back to the same color?**
Not immediately. As with any teeth whitening product when you stop using it your teeth may over time become less white particularly if you drink soda or coffee or smoke. If you notice your teeth becoming yellower you can simply use the activated charcoal powder again to brighten them.

**How long does the activated charcoal powder last?**
This depends on the size of the product you order. In general a 2 OZ jar could last as many as 2-3 months for one person. Remember, you should use very little powder each time you brush – with activated charcoal powder a little goes a long way.

**Will activated charcoal stain my sink?**
If you thoroughly rinse and wipe down the sink after using the activated charcoal it should not stain.

**Is activated charcoal safe for your enamel?**
Be sure to brush normally or gently when using the activated charcoal to help protect your enamel.

**Are the results permanent?**
No. While the whitening results may last longer than some other methods eventually your teeth may darken depending on what you eat or drink and you will need to again use the activated charcoal powder to brighten them. This process is the same for all teeth whitening products.

**How often should I use activated charcoal?**
This is up to you. You can use it once a day or twice a day or a few times a week or month – it really is up to you and what you want to achieve. When your teeth reach a certain level of whiteness you may then want to use it once a week or as needed to keep your teeth from getting yellower.

**Can I use activated charcoal with braces?**

We recommend waiting until your braces are removed to prevent havi
yellow spots on your teeth where your braces were.

**Is activated charcoal OK to use on sensitive teeth?**

Yes, you can use most activated charcoal formulas on sensitive teeth.

**Will activated charcoal make my teeth more sensitive?**

If used properly, it shouldn't. Brush gently and use it for 1 to 2 minut
then rinse thoroughly.

**How white will activated charcoal make my teeth?**

This varies by individual. Some experience excellent results with activa
ed charcoal powder while others see less dramatic improvement.

**Can I use activated charcoal powder everyday or is there a lin
it?**

There is no limit, you can use it as much as you want to brighten ar
clean your teeth. Many use it twice a day. Plus, it really helps get rid
bad breath – along with plaque.

**Does activated charcoal harm the gums?**

No, it removes plaque which helps the gums. Activated charcoal is al
easier on the gums than many other whitening products which conta
chemicals and can cause burning.

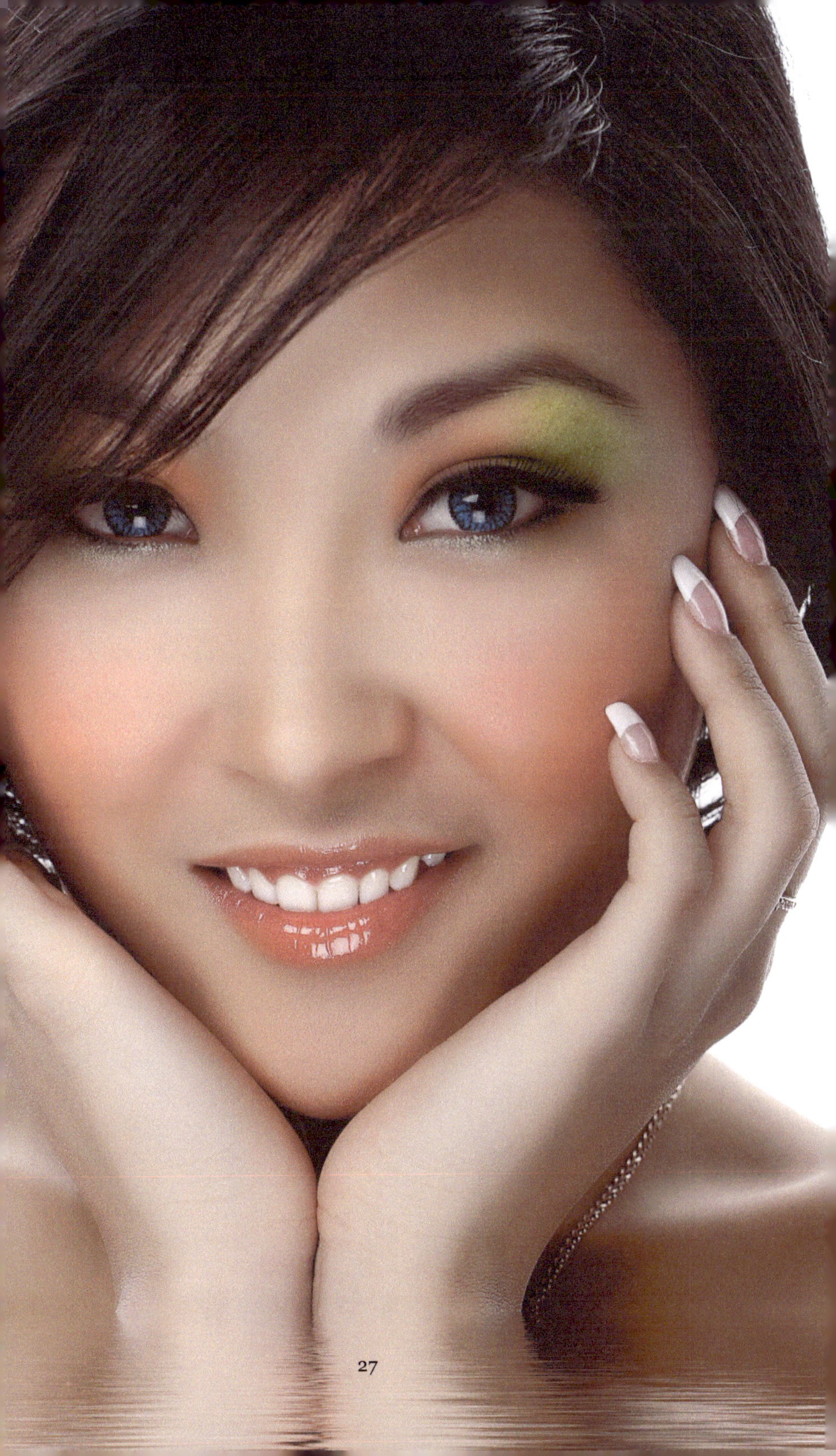

# How to Keep Your New Smile White

You must first recognize and minimize the culprits that could be staining your teeth.

If you are a foodie like me, you tend to think more about how food affects your figure more than the little things like how certain foods can stain your teeth. But if you want to look good from head to toe, you should be aware of these common foods and drinks that could be staining your teeth:

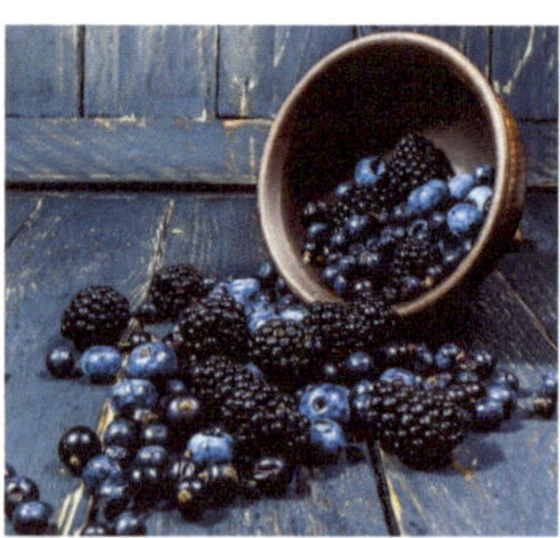

- Cherries
- Pomegranate
- Blueberries
- Blackberries
- Cranberries
- Beets
- Curry

> **REMEMBER THIS TIP**: *"If your food or beverage will stain a white t-shirt, think twice because it could also potentially stain your teeth!"* - **Dr. Catrise Austin**

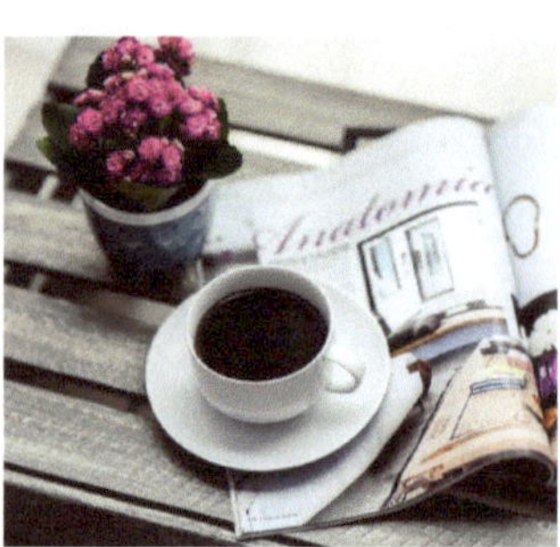

- Red Wine
- Coffee & Tea
- Balsamic Vinegar
- Dark Cola
- Soy, Worchestire, and Steak Sauces
- Tomato-based Sauces and More!

To keep your new smile white, make sure brush and rinse or your teeth as soon as possible after consuming the above foods.

## Daily Oral Care: Brush, Floss, Rinse.

Keeping your smile also requires you to be diligent with your daily oral hygiene. Here's what I want you all to do, follow the simple steps of my smile workout every day:

1. Brush
2. Floss
3. Rinse

### *Brush for 2 minutes 3 times a day*

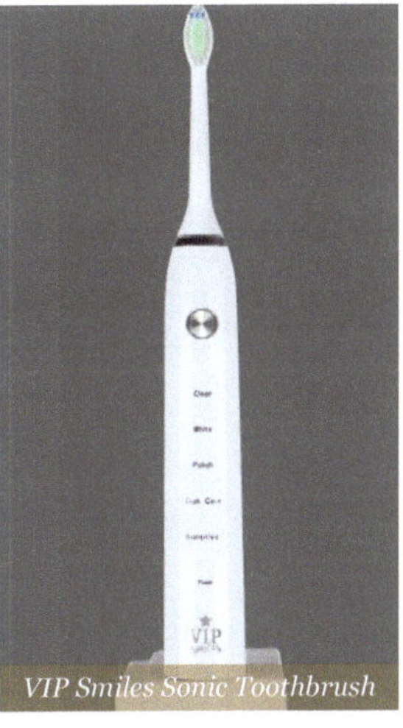

VIP Smiles Sonic Toothbrush

Brush for 2 whole minutes or break that down into 30 secs for each section of your mouth with a sonic toothbrush or soft manual toothbrush.

If using a regular tooth brush, I suggest you use one with soft bristles (such as the VIP Smiles bamboo soft toothbrush) as medium or hard can lead to enamel wear and sensitivity over time.

As another option, I highly recommend sonic toothbrushes for teeth whitening maintenance. They are the way to go for preventing and removing stains! Combine the sonic toothbrush with your favorite whitening toothpaste and your smile will sparkle for the long haul.

Our VIP Smiles sonic toothbrush vibrates at 40,000 brush strokes per minute, 9,000 more than the leading sonic brand. As a point of comparison, conventional electric toothbrushes generate 2,500 to 7,500 strokes-per-minute.

Why is it important to have 40,000 brush strokes per minute? Because this brush head speed creates a secondary cleansing action (fluid dynamics) that gets rid of plaque beyond where the bristles can reach.

That's right, our sonic toothbrush helps you get rid of more harmful plaque through fluid dynamics, which is the process by which the brush speed agitates saliva and water in the mouth causing it to disrupt plaque that brush bristles can't get to.

## Next, Floss Daily

This is where most people blow it!!! Floss at least 2 times daily between your teeth to remove plaque and prevent the formation of tartar between the teeth. Tartar turns tan or brown over time and picks up stains easily which can quickly ruin the color of your teeth.

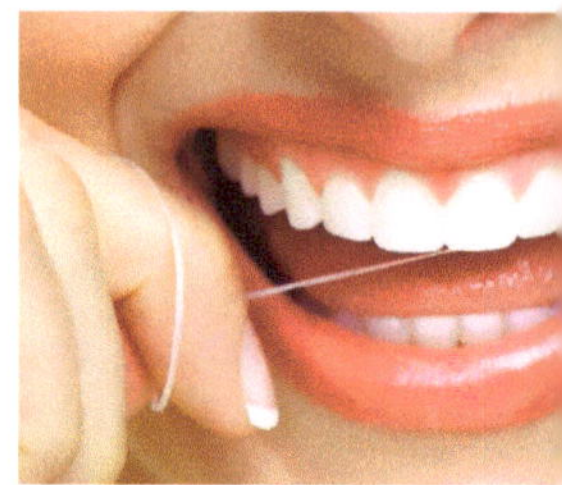

I love those pre-loaded floss picks that come in a bag of 75 or 100, it makes flossing so easy! If you just can't get into the rhythm of flossing manually, I highly recommend using a water flosser like WaterPik. It's like a carwash for your mouth! Use the hose to blast plaque and stains from your teeth. You may find it less tedious than manual flossing.

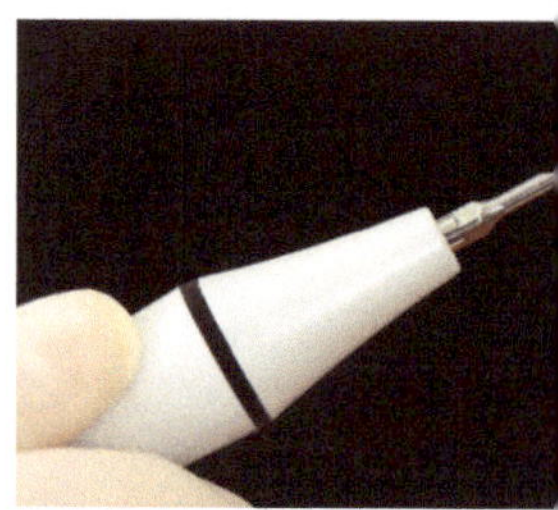

## Rinse

If you enjoy foods and drinks that stain your teeth, always follow them with a glass of water. To keep stain causing dyes and bacteria from sticking to your teeth at home, choose an alcohol free or whitening mouthwash for maintenance.

Always on the go? Make sure to travel size it! Always be armed to fight stains by carrying travel sized toothbrush, toothpaste, mouthwash. These are great tools to use to protect your smile throughout the day.

## Chew On This!

### Chewing gum

Not only are there whitening gums on the market today, but ANY chewing gum increases the flow of saliva, which works to eat away at the stains on your teeth.

## Go Raw

While chewing gum creates saliva, so does chewing raw crunchy foods like carrots, apples, celery, broccoli, cauliflower. Not only are these raw fruits and vegetables nutritional, but chewing on them will stimulate more saliva which can naturally aid in keeping the stains from sticking to your teeth.

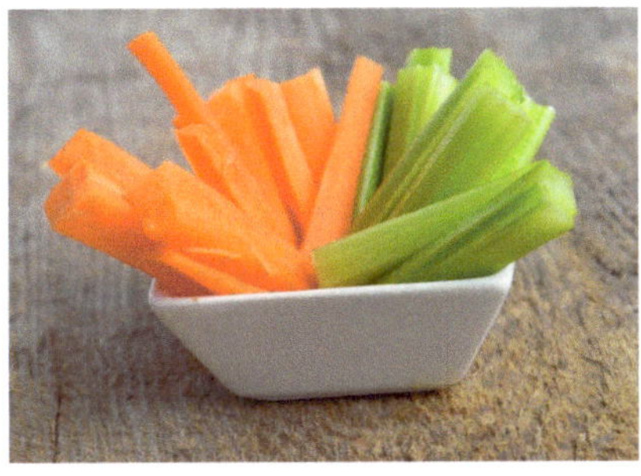

### *Take A Few Extra Trips to the Dentist*

Most patients can control stains and keep their teeth relatively clean and white between their normal every 6 month dental office visits by practicing good oral hygiene habits at home. However if you notice that your teeth stain or build up tartar quickly, you may need to increase

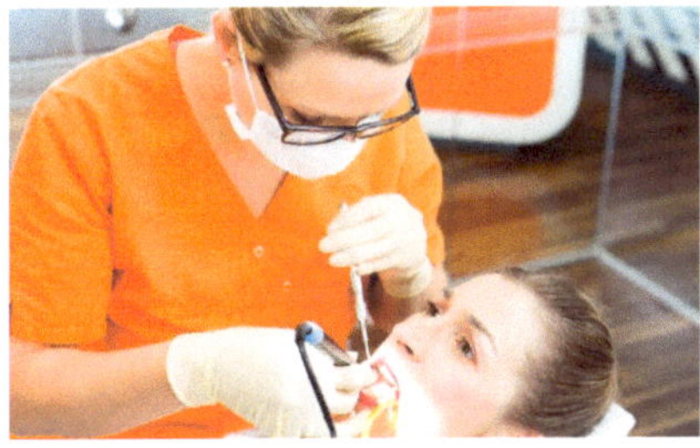

your visits to the dentist from every 6 months to every 3-4 months to have your teeth professionally cleaned. Although these extra teeth cleanings may not be covered by your dental insurance, it will be worth the investment to let the pro's help keep you white!

### *Suck It!*

When drinking your favorite dark colored beverages, a straw can be your secret weapon! Drinking through a straw allows the stain-causing dyes to bypass the teeth, keeping your smile brighter much longer. Many celebrities, such as Justin Bieber and Miley Cyrus, use this technique! So next time you need your coffee or tea fix, try the iced versions – and drink them with a straw.

# More Natural Home Remedies for a Whiter Smile

You don't always have to pay for whiter teeth! If times are tough and every penny counts or you enjoy trying natural remedies, in this section I will share a few recipes that can help. These natural teeth whitening pastes and rinses are not only chemical-free, but they are literally FREE! The great thing is that many of the items used in these recipes can be found in your cupboard, pantry, fridge or medicine cabinet at this very moment. Unlike the peroxide-based whitening products on the market, these natural remedies won't eliminate the deep internal stains from your teeth, but will help remove plaque and stains from the outer enamel to make them shine brighter.

**Caution:** Some of the following recipes call for the use of acidic fruits which are not meant to be applied daily. Use them sparingly, no more than once a week to avoid side effects of tooth erosion or tooth sensitivity.

## Fresh Strawberries

It's rumored that Catherine Zeta-Jones uses strawberries to keep her teeth lustrous and white. True or not, research has proven that the malic acid in a single strawberry can reduce stains associated with coffee and tea.

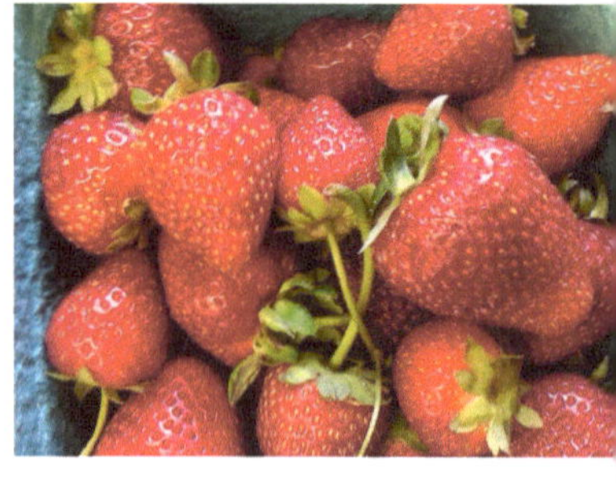

Just cut a strawberry and rub the fresh strawberry across each tooth as you might a toothbrush for 2 minutes. Then brush and rinse like you routinely do with toothpaste and water to make sure to eliminate residual acid from strawberries.

## Homemade Baking Soda Whitening Toothpaste

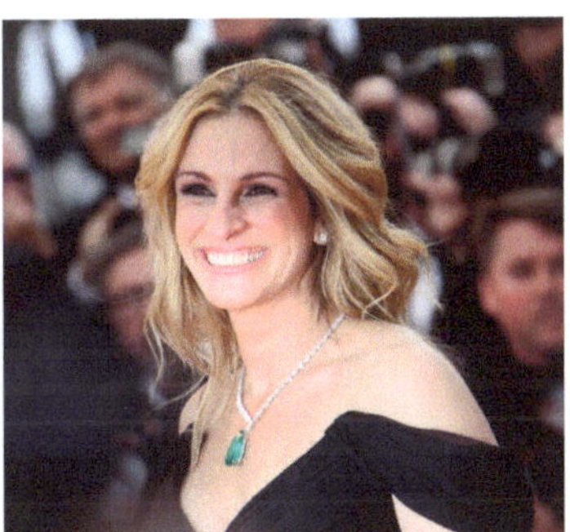
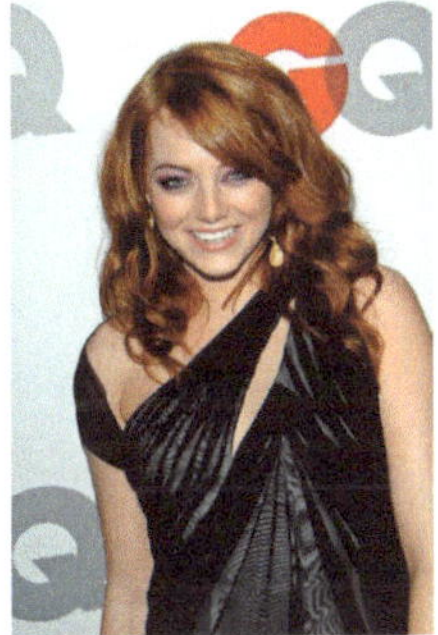
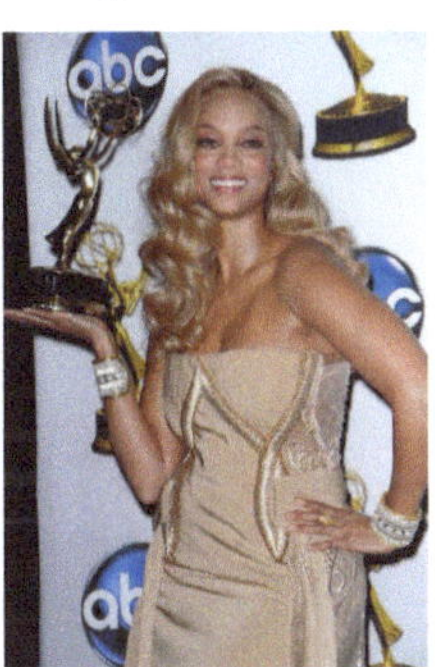

Julia Roberts, Emma Stone, Queen Latifah and Tyra Banks are known to use baking soda to keep their teeth white. Here's an old school whitening trick that I bet even your grandparents tried back in the day!

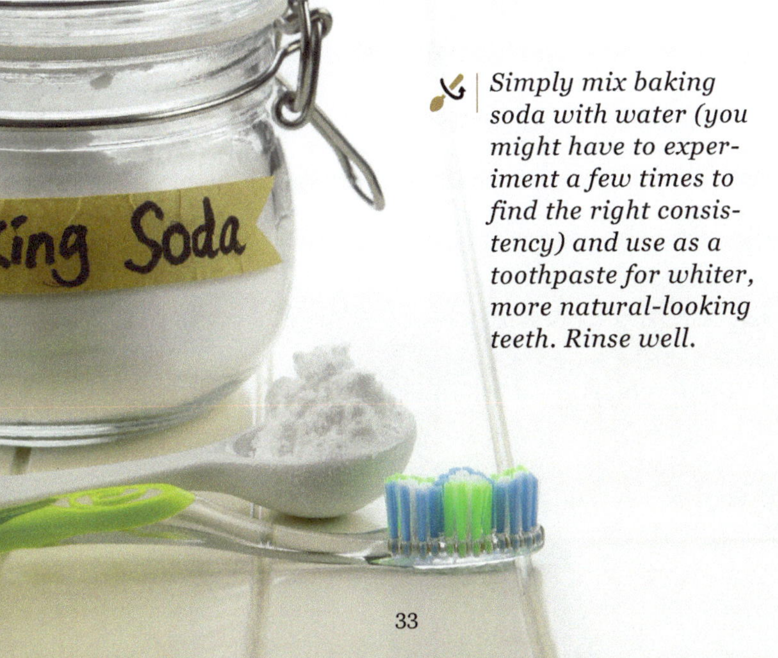

*Simply mix baking soda with water (you might have to experiment a few times to find the right consistency) and use as a toothpaste for whiter, more natural-looking teeth. Rinse well.*

Warning: Baking soda is abrasive. If you use baking soda too often, the enamel on your teeth can become damaged. I recommend using this no more than once a week.

# Homemade Strawberry Whitening Toothpaste

You can also combine the strawberry and baking soda recipes to create strawberry toothpaste! This recipe calls for both strawberries and baking soda to make a fruity tasting paste that can brighten your smile.

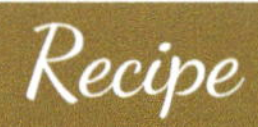

**INGREDIENTS:**

- 1 medium mixing bowl
- 1 fork
- 1 large strawberry
- 1/2 Tsp of Baking Soda

**DIRECTIONS:**

*Take 1 large strawberry and cut off the stem. In a medium mixing bowl, crush the strawberry using a fork until it is a mush consistency. Next, add 1/2 Tsp of Baking Soda to the crushed strawberry and mix together well.*

**FROM THE KITCHEN OF** *Dr. Catrise Aus*

# Hydrogen Peroxide Whitening Mouthwash

Gargling with hydrogen peroxide is also known to brighten teeth. This true to some extent, but keep in mind that over-the-counter hydrogen peroxide is not nearly as concentrated as that found in professional teeth whiteners. Whitening with hydrogen peroxide is safe as long as you dilute it and also don't swallow it.

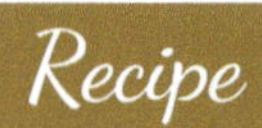

**INGREDIENTS:**

- 3 Tbsp Hydrogen peroxide
- 1 Tbsp water
- 1 mason jar or cup

**DIRECTIONS:**

*Try mixing three parts hydrogen peroxide and one part water to reduce the potency of the peroxide, which in turn reduces your chance of experiencing tooth and gum sensitivity.*

**FROM THE KITCHEN OF** *Dr. Catrise Aus*

# Kicked-Up Strawberry Whitening Toothpaste

If you like strawberries, here's a kicked-up version of the strawberry teeth whitening toothpaste. This recipe calls for using fresh strawberries and baking soda, but this time you can take it to the next level by adding hydrogen peroxide!

**INGREDIENTS:**
- 1 medium mixing bowl
- 1 fork
- 1 large strawberry
- 2-3 Tsp of Baking Soda
- 2-3 Tsp of Peroxide

***DIRECTIONS:***
*Take 1 large strawberry and cut off the stem. In a medium mixing bowl, crush the strawberry using a fork until it is a mushy consistency. Next, add 1/2 Tsp of Baking Soda to the crushed strawberry. This time add 2-3 Tsp of peroxide and mix together well.*

**FROM THE KITCHEN OF** *Dr. Catrise Austin*

# Baking Soda Dipped Whitening Toothpaste

Here's another baking soda trick that will keep your smile whiter!

**INGREDIENTS:**
- 1 Colgate Optic White Toothpaste
- 1 Colgate 360 soft toothbrush or Electric toothbrush
- 1/2 Tsp of Baking Soda

***DIRECTIONS:***
*Using a soft manual toothbrush or an electric toothbrush, place the desired amount of whitening toothpaste on the brush. Simply dip your toothbrush in baking soda to capture a nice amount of baking soda and brush.*

**FROM THE KITCHEN OF** *Dr. Catrise Austin*

# Zesty Fresh Orange Flavored
# Whitening Toothpaste

Many people swear by this simple and zesty recipe!

### INGREDIENTS:

- 1 medium storage bowl with lid
- 1 hand shredder
- 1 mixer or food processor
- 1 large orange
- 1/2 Tsp of Baking Soda
- 1-2 Tsp of Peroxide

*DIRECTIONS:*

*Orange rinds can also be ground into a so_ fine, orange-ish powder along with baki_ soda and salt in a food processor. Stored_ an airtight container and mixed with a ti_ amount of hydrogen peroxide, this natur_ remedy makes for a great teeth whitener._*

FROM THE KITCHEN OF *Dr. Catrise Aus_*

You can also take the inside of an orange rind and rub it against your tee_ for brighter, whiter teeth without chemicals or dentist visits.

# Fresh Lemon Flavored
# Whitening Rinse

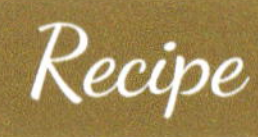

### INGREDIENTS:

- 3 Tbsp Fresh lemon juice
- 1 Tbsp salt
- 1 cup of water

*DIRECTIONS:*

*Blend the three ingredients together. Y_ can use them as a mouthwash of sor_ swishing it around for a minute or so befo_ spitting it out, then rinsing thoroughly a_ brushing your teeth as usual. This meth_ also promotes gum health._*

FROM THE KITCHEN OF *Dr. Catrise Aus_*

Mixing three parts fresh lemon juice (3 tablespoons) to one part salt (1 t_ blespoon) has long been a favorite home remedy for whiter teeth witho_ bleach or gels. Once the two ingredients are blended together, you can u_ them as a mouthwash of sorts, swishing it around for a minute or so befo_ spitting it out, then rinsing thoroughly and brushing your teeth as usu_ This method also promotes gum health.

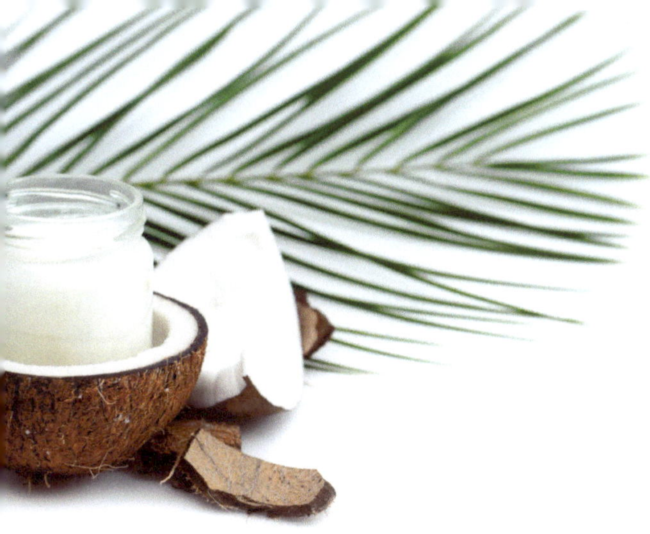

## Coconut Oil

Over the past 2 years I've had many clients ask me about the recent craze of oil pulling!  Oil pulling is an ancient dental technique that has been revived that involves swishing your mouth with coconut oil.  With its natural antibiotic and anti-viral properties, oil pulling has not only been alleged to reduce the amount of harmful bacteria in your mouth but also brightens your teeth. Celebrities such as Bella Thorne, Vanessa Hudgens, Leigh-Anne Pinnock, Louise Thompson, Ashley Benson, Charlotte Crosby, Lindsay Lohan, Gwyneth Paltrow and Shailene Woodley are said to use oil pulling to whiten their teeth.

You'll need:

1 Tbsp. of Extra Virgin Organic Cold Pressed Coconut Oil. Trader Joe's, Whole Foods and other stores now sell coconut oil.

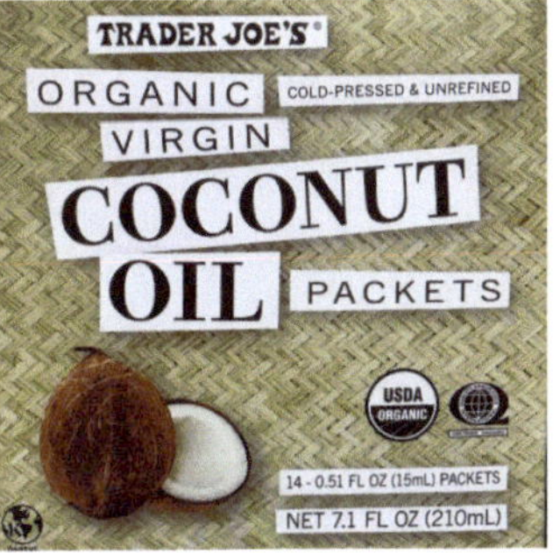


Here's how it works:  Use 1 Tbsp. of coconut oil and swish it around your mouth for 5-20 minutes, then spit it out.  Be careful not to swallow the oil! Next, brush your teeth and rinse your mouth to remove any residual coconut oil.  That's it.  Try this for up to 2 weeks and those who have tried it swear that it does wonders.

**Caution:** It's been suggested by both the American Dental Association (ADA) and the U.S. Department of Health and Humans Services that the practice of oil-pulling has not been extensively tested and proven to have dental benefits. If you decide to give it a try however, rinsing your mouth with coconut oil probably will not cause any harm as long as you keep up a good dental care routine and whitening results can't be guaranteed to make your teeth whiter.

## Sage

Native Americans are said to have used sage to both freshen breath and whiten their teeth.

Use fresh sage leaves and, as with orange rind and strawberries, simply rub them against your teeth for fresher breath and whiter teeth instantly.

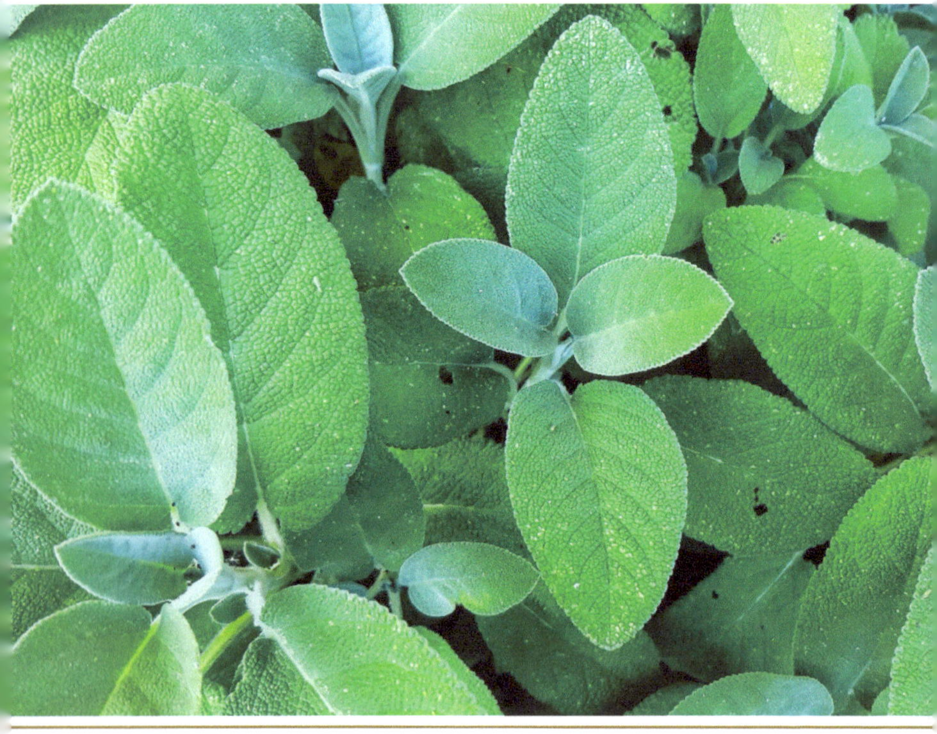

# Conclusion

If you are OK with seeing your teeth and gums temporarily turn black while brushing with activated charcoal this can be a very effective way to get rid of surface stains and whiten your teeth.

As we stated previously, activated charcoal is less expensive than many other whitening methods and can work just as well. It can also be gentler on the gums than whitening treatments that contain chemicals.

Just remember that activated charcoal can be messy. So you will want to use it cautiously. It can also be difficult to remove from your mouth. We recommend brushing with toothpaste and flossing afterwards to ensure you get rid of all the charcoal particles.

Those, in a nutshell, are the pluses and minuses of using activated charcoal. If, after reading this book, you feel that this treatment is right for you, we highly recommend **VIP Smiles Organic Coconut Charcoal Teeth Whitening Powder**.

This powder is 2 FL OZ Food Grade Activated Charcoal which brightens teeth, is easy on the gums, is mint flavored and has no bad after-taste.

You can learn much more about this amazing product by visiting www.vipsmilesstore.com

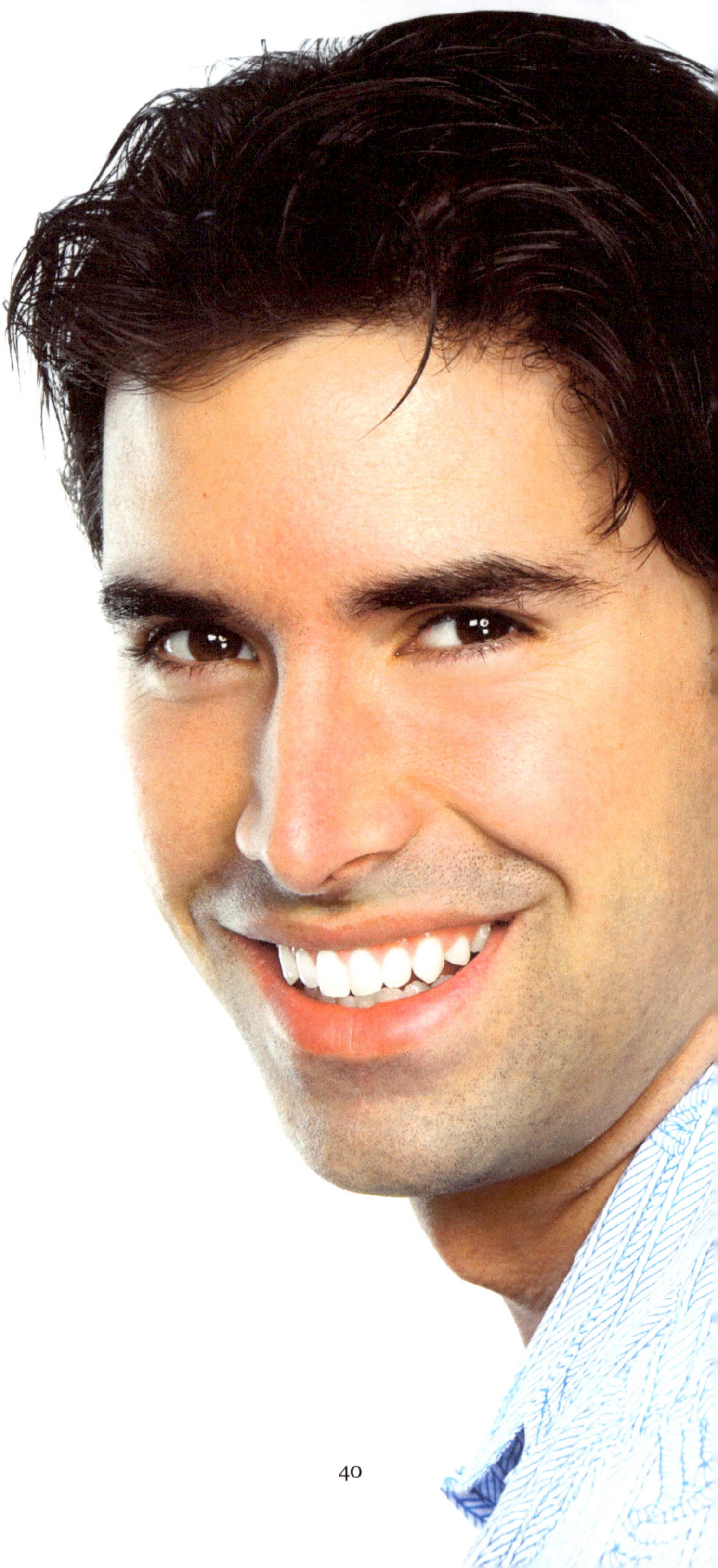

# About the Author

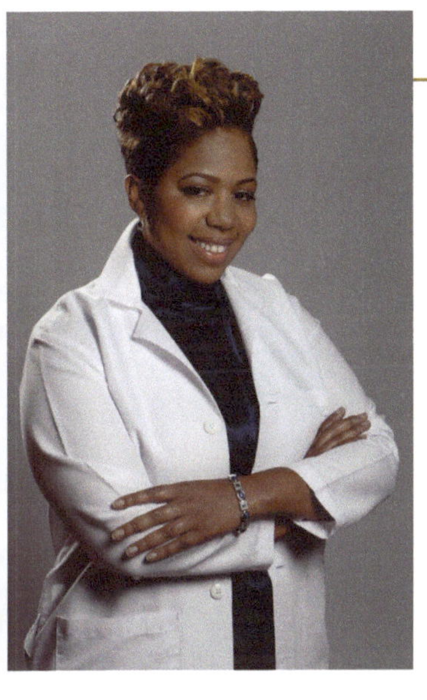

For 20 years now, cosmetic dentist Dr. Catrise Austin, known as The Queen of Smiles, has been in the business of transforming smiles for singles, business people, celebrities, and anyone looking to simply enjoy life with a better smile.

With hard work, and despite many odds, this Flint, Michigan native not only has been named as one of the "Top 25 Women In Dentistry", she's been a featured cosmetic dentistry expert on NBC's Today Show, ABC News in Chicago and Reno, and even TMZ.

In 2017, her national media book tour allowed her to share smile makeover tips from her #1 international bestseller book called "GetSmiled: The Ultimate Guide To Improving Your Image With Your Greatest Asset—Your Smile!". She was also invited to be a featured speaker at The Harvard Faculty Club in Cambridge where she shared the stage with health and business mogul Suzanne Somers and was presented an award for her speech on "The Power Of A Smile" in business.

Consumer studies conducted on behalf of The American Academy of Cosmetic Dentistry (AACD) have proved that having a beautiful smile will not only make you more attractive, but will make you appear more intelligent, interesting, successful, and wealthy to others as well.

Dr. Catrise Austin recently got a chance to test this theory out when she was called by the popular VH1 reality TV show Love and Hip Hop New York to transform the smile of its breakout star rapper Cardi B.

Cardi B had been constantly ridiculed on social media about her less tha
perfect smile. In just 2 short visits, Dr. Austin transformed Cardi B's smi
with teeth whitening and porcelain veneers and literally changed her life.

When the transformation debuted on the season premiere episode of Lov
and Hip Hop New York in November 2016, it sparked a smile makeov
frenzy!
The newfound confidence from her new smile led Cardi B to rap about h
smile transformation on her #1 Billboard song "Bodak Yellow". Now Dr. C
trise Austin is living her dreams by helping consumers from all over th
world inspired by Cardi B to "GetSmiled" by The Queen of Smiles.

The best has yet to come from Dr. Austin in 2018. This year she has reache
another goal by launching her own brand of affordable teeth whitenin
products called "VIP Smiles by Dr. Catrise Austin."

She believes that having a beautiful and confident smile is not just a luxur
it is a necessity!

With these new cosmetic dentistry products available at www.vipsmiles
tore.com she hopes to give consumers all over the world a chance to tal
their smiles to the next level and look like a million bucks, for less.

Dr. Austin is showing no signs of slowing down this year as she'll be spea
ing at Coca Cola and Harvard, releasing 2 more books, launching live sem
nars, and making more TV appearances nation-wide.

Keep up with Dr. Catrise Austin by following her @drcatriseaustin on soci
media!